My gift

to help you

quit smoking

Why I started to smoke cigarettes and
how I liberated myself from the tobacco addiction.
Stop smoking and stay nicotine free!

Peter Kruse

NOTES OF THANKS

Cherie Fox for the great cover
www.cheriefox.com

Katherine Wadkins and Terry Kenworthy
for proofreading

Matthias Rost for his professional guidance as an
experienced addiction counselor

Dr. Horst Freels and Psychologist Maria Eugenia
Diaz for the medical and psychological expertise

My test readers for their valuable feedback

***

Dedicated to my daughters
Monica & Lessa Belle

CONTENT

"People do not smoke cigarettes.
Cigarettes smoke people."

(Manfred Hinrich)

FOREWORD BY MATTHIAS ROST

"To stop smoking is dead easy. I managed to do it more than a hundred times already." (Mark Twain)

To quit smoking – this is a thought every smoker has had at least once. Whether through his own initiative or because friends or a doctor suggests it. Somehow, it's very clear in the back of their mind – one day I will quit. Just… maybe not today. Perhaps when I am 30/50/70 years old, or when I face lung cancer/whooping cough/COPD etc. Or maybe when cigarettes cost 10€/20€/30€ a pack. One of these days, I will quit.

Dear reader, have you ever had these kinds of thoughts yourself? Then you have found the right book. This book is not a panacea. There is no such thing. It is the critical self-reflection of an ex-smoker. It is open, honest and direct.

Some will shake their heads and keep smoking as before. Others may smile, feel a bit guilty, but still not change anything. But maybe – *maybe* one thought or another will remain stuck and will lead suddenly to the conclusion, that it is very rewarding indeed, to ban the glowing slave master from its own life.

Smoking remains the number one avoidable cause of death. In Germany 330 people die daily of the consequences of consumption of tobacco. That would be like a fully loaded Boeing 777 crashing somewhere in our country every day. But why is it so hard to talk about it?

Well, in fact, each year the German government does publish the statistics of drug related death rates. Unfortunately though, these figures only include people who died from the consumption of *illegal* drugs. And every time these numbers are shocking, because it is a total of around 1,300 persons... per year. The number of casualties through tobacco will thus exceed this figure already on 5th of January of every year. Yes, we as a society have wonderfully managed to fade out the real problem.

Therefore, dear reader. Please remain critical and accept that you may feel uneasy at some passages of this book. I can assure you that it is not due to the book. It may be because your head tries to unite the new thoughts with your life so far. Somehow, these considerations do not fit together. It may be rather uncomfortable at first – but perhaps it is the first step towards a new life.

Yes, the best moment for this step may have been 5/10/20 or more years ago, but the second best moment is **today**!

Quitting smoking is easy. The difficult part is not to start again.

Matthias Rost
Social Pedagogue/Addiction Therapist -
Diakonie Leipzig/Germany

PROLOG

"Do you want to give up smoking? Perhaps you would like to help me. I just wrote a book about my experiences of how I became a happy nonsmoker after 40 years of considering myself an enjoyable smoker. Before publishing, I would like to find out if, and how well, my book and the method I have used will work with others.

Are you a SMOKER? Do you want to seriously quit smoking for good?

If yes, then please text me a personal message. I would love to send you the script and receive your observations.

I am looking forward to hearing from you…"

This ad appeared in the Facebook groups "Test readers required", "Search and find test readers", as well as in different groups about non-smoking.

The feedback from over one hundred volunteers who contacted me, mostly heavy smokers, made it possible to write this book the way it is. It allowed me to rethink the script and include/exclude aspects, which I would not have considered without the valuable comments, suggestions and experiences shared by my test readers

For forty years of my life, I considered myself a committed and passionate smoker. One package per day was typical, but quite often it was even more, depending on the circumstances and my mood. Every smoker knows what I am talking about.

Smoking was cool when I started… that is what I thought, and why I did it.

My simple motto was:

"The one who smokes, dies. The one, who does not smoke, also dies. So just enjoy life as long as you can."

I was firmly convinced that consumption of tobacco:

✓ gave me pleasure
✓ relaxed me
✓ increased my concentration
✓ kept me awake
✓ made me more sociable
✓ gave me self-assurance
✓ was cool
✓ etc.

Then, one fine day, as a consequence of a very unexpected medical diagnose, I realized that my life motto, in itself, was quite ok. However, the connection with cigarettes was self-delusional. It was horrendous nonsense! I suddenly realized how I had cheated myself by assigning attributes to tobacco consumption that are simply not applicable. I understood that day, that I had betrayed myself for forty years, just so I could indulge my smoking desire without developing a bad conscience.

The results and consequences of smoking had been completely misinterpreted. I let myself fantasize that the obvious disadvantages would be alleged advantages. I was brainwashed.

Luckily, that time has finally ended. Today, a cigarette is about as appealing to me as a hearty swig of warm cod liver oil. Zero desire, zero attraction!

"To quit a habit is purely a matter of willpower. You just have to be fully convinced and strong, and then you can do it"

How many times have we heard this assertion, and confirmed it with an affirmative nod of the head? But it is only half the truth. This thesis only applies to habits we do not want to break. But, if it comes in handy, then one is very well able to discard any custom in a flash and without major mental effort.

To get up at 6 am, to torture oneself with the bus to work, to live alone and to do the same boring job are all habits we grudgingly accept. How incredibly fast does each of us suddenly get used to getting up at 8 am, driving to work in a brand new car, finding love and taking on a more attractive job? Yes, these changes of habit take place in record time. Even those who, for the last five years, have been bored of doing the same laps in the prison yard get used to walking straight ahead, jumping and running in freedom in no time.

The relativity of the habits is even evident in smokers themselves. The vast majority of female ex-smokers report how effortlessly they managed to quit smoking after finding out that they were pregnant. Even though it had seemed to be almost impossible for them, before.

So the whole truth is that each of us is quite capable of changing habits easily and quickly. It is only ever considered difficult or impossible by us humans if we feel the change to be negative or do not want to do it. This is the reason why the smoker always complains. All he has to do is recognize the habit of smoking for what it is... a completely unnecessary and annoying action. Then it will be just as easy for him to give up this routine in the future.

My first step towards finally becoming a non-smoker was to have serious thoughts about why all my previous attempts had been unsuccessful. I concluded that they were all based on willpower, so what went wrong?

As a result of my brainstorming, emerged the approach that eventually worked, so easily and pleasantly for me. This is what I want so share and what this book is about.

Like many other smokers too, I also needed several attempts before I finally found the right method that worked for me. When I did, though, it was suddenly surprisingly simple, to say good-bye to the smokestack. Almost like from one moment to the next. The feeling was equally nice as unbelievable. Before, I always felt that renouncing my beloved vice would be a torture.

In order to give the "baby" a name, I call my successfully exercised procedure the **"Lead-motive method"**. It's based on a behavioral theory that I studied as a young man, long ago, while attending university. With the "Lead-motive method", my final farewell from tobacco was neither difficult nor related to a feeling of loss. On the contrary, this time I literally enjoyed the jump into a smoke free life, from the last cigarette onwards. I had no noteworthy withdrawal symptoms, no major side effects, and no struggle with myself. From the very first day on, I realized that it would be plain easy. And so it was.

Night after night, I went to sleep with the pleasant feeling of not having touched a steaming coffin nail for another whole day. Not even the slightest need arose in me. In the mornings, I woke up with a smile and was proud of myself. I felt fresh and healthy, without the craving for my "artist's breakfast" (coffee and a hand rolled cigarette), that I had practiced daily for decades.

Now, being a non-smoker, I enjoy the aroma of a cup of good coffee every time I get up, without puffing at the same time. After 40 years of numbed taste buds, I had completely forgotten what coffee enjoyment means. Simply divine. Suddenly I drank it black, without sugar and milk. Just so as not to lose the true charm of the coffee bean. Smoke and soot had numbed my sense of taste over the years to such an extent that I could no longer consciously perceive what a delicacy I was consuming. Not only with coffee, but also with everything else I ate and drank. Without having consciously planned it, all my previous eating habits changed little by little, as I could taste again, what I drank, chewed, or swallowed.

My second life, that of the pleasurable non-smoker, began when I became aware that I only have one life. After the aforementioned medical diagnosis, the rock-solid will to delightfully enjoy every further day of the rest of my life became anchored in me. Not damage to health was the driving force. It was the rediscovered world of real enjoyment. Luckily, it is never too late for starting something better.

In this booklet, I would like to pass on my experiences to all those who have not yet reached their goal because they have taken the difficult path. What I have to tell is surprisingly simple and has worked for me without major problems or difficulties. Because yes, sometimes a book helps you understand what is going on inside yourself.

Please do not worry if you have not completely lost all desire for a cigarette right after the first ten pages of this book. A little patience is needed. I can assure you, the doubt will not last for very long. All people who start smoking need a certain amount of time before they think they like the taste of a cigarette. For most people, it will be a similar experience when they quit. But believe me, in my experience, it will only be a short period before you can be sure that burnt tobacco tastes awful in your mouth.

Even if only one person gives up smoking using the method in this book, it would be a success, because I might have saved someone from a terrible illness. I hope that it is exactly YOU who I could help. Then that makes us already two happy people.

"Fortunately, the caterpillar did not give up. Just when he thought he would never make it, he started to fly."

Some of the data and information given at the beginning of this book may already be familiar to you. For those readers who are quitting smoking for the first time, and who have not read anything or very little about it, it serves to increase awareness. For everyone else, they are useful refreshers of important facts. Repetition is one of the cornerstones of the method I present. You will therefore read some of the most relevant points several times.

I do not claim that the reading of this book will bear fruit for everyone. Nobody ever managed this nor will most probably anybody ever do. A book can only help, if the reader is willing and ready to accept it. I studied business administration in Germany, as well as marketing and philosophy in England. I am not an addiction researcher, nor have I done any studies or collected statistics. I just want to report how I achieved success and freedom personally.

"I did it my way." I am not selling a universal cure-all.

But in my life, so far I have made the astonishing discovery that you can learn something from everyone, no matter whether it is a proven expert or an amateur. Even from whom you would not consider clever at first glance. The only important thing is the willingness to open your ears. In this sense, I hope that one or the other smoker will benefit from my story. As this is a personal perspective, you may not agree with everything I say, but it can still work if you just focus on what convinces you.

If you find something you like while reading, please take a short break at that point. Let what you have read sink in and anchor within yourself. I suggest you keep a highlighter or pencil handy. As soon as you discover a text passage where you think "yes, that's right, that's true", you should mark it.

Now I wish you a lot of pleasure while reading and hopefully the success you dream for. Make yourself comfortable, light a "tasty" cigarette with "pleasure" and start reading. The "worst" thing that can happen to you is that, at the end of the book, you will no longer feel like smoking.

20 minutes after your last cigarette:
Pulse and blood pressure are beginning to normalize

SUDDENLY SILENT

"Really? Well, and how do you explain then that Grandpa Ghoto got to be over 100 years old even though he smoked like a chimney, you wise guy?"

"And Winston Churchill, remember? He turned 90 years by smoking at least 10 cigars every day."

With these kinds of examples, all of which smokers love to quote, I had so far silenced every well-meaning health apostle. Even now, my well intentioned friend had to admit that smoking apparently does not, in all cases, necessarily lead to an early death. Sensing his insecurity, a self-satisfied smile spread across my face as I skillfully fished a cigarette out of the leather case and lit it with relish. Once again, I had won.

"Well then, do what you want" was his response.

"Yes, that's exactly what I'm going to do", I said. *"You only live once and why should I give up something I enjoy? I am not an altar boy. He, who has no vice, does not have a longer life… it just seems longer to him, hahahahahha.".*

Boom! Another low blow to the boring moralist. No, I did not want anyone to spoil my smoking pleasure that easily. My self-created philosophy was: If you enjoy the cigarette, it will not harm you. Only those who smoke with a guilty conscience, who regret every cigarette in their soul as soon as they light it, will be affected. Any damage caused by smoking was, in my naïve view, psychosomatically caused. I was convinced that only the permanent strain on the soul leads to physical impairment. Since I was guilt free, I was sure that nothing could happen to me.

Oh yes, I was one of those. I saw myself as a pleasure smoker who would easily pass the 100 years mark. One, of whom all dangers simply bounce off, ... I was invulnerable.

Then, I received the diagnose: bladder tumor.

> *"Cancer?"* I asked the urologist.
> *"I'm sorry to have to tell you,"* he nodded.
> *"Why? Where does it come from?"*
> *"Do you smoke,"* he asked me.

Grandpa Ghoto and Winston Churchill had suddenly become small and quiet in my head. The arrogance evaporated. I had finally understood: **Smoking is no fun!** Yes, it is true. There are heavy smokers who reach an advanced age. There are also people who hit the jackpot in the lottery. Nevertheless, I have never personally met any of these "lucky devils". They are a tiny minority. Therefore, one should be careful with the assumption that one will always be on the winning side.

No nicotine addict automatically drops dead after consuming a certain number of smoked cigarettes. If this were the case, all but the outright suicidal would stop just short of this last possible moment. The Grandpa Ghotos and the Winston Churchills of this world therefore suggest the illusion "nothing will happen to me". I, too, was so arrogant and so boastful about my smoking.

Not an early death should be chosen as a criterion on which to make smoking or non-smoking dependent. Death is as much a part of life as birth even though we humans tend to suppress it from our everyday thoughts. Both things happen. More important than *when*, for most people, is *how* they will die. And there is no doubt that smokers have an extremely good chance of spending the last part of their lives in great agony. At the latest on their deathbed, however, I am convinced that every smoker will whisper to you *"do not be stupid like me... do not smoke!"*

More decisive is the lung cancer possibly diagnosed one day (90% of all lung cancer patients are smokers), impotence (twice as often as with non-smokers) or early heart and circulation problems, as highly probable consequences of smoking. With every intake of smoking poison, inhaled hour after hour, day after day, we play a risky game with our body and we lose quality of life. In my case, it was "just" a bladder tumor. My cancer did not spread. It was detected and removed in time. My life goes on. My smoking does not!

Still, what are we going to do with our highly quoted Grandpa Ghoto? Well, that fellow is simply a phenomenon in many ways. The exception to the rule that always exists and for which no one seems to know the explanation.

12 hours after his last cigarette:

All organs receive a better oxygen supply

THE OTHER DAY AT THE
PATENT OFFICE

"Yes?"

"Mr. Marlboro is waiting outside."

"Have him come in."

"Good afternoon, Mr. Marlboro. Please be seated. What can I do for you?"

"Thank you very much. I have come to file a patent application for my invention."

"Very well, what is it about?"

"My invention is called 'cigarette'. It is something completely new, unprecedented and revolutionary. Soon millions of people will not be able to imagine how life was possible before, without my product."

"That sounds very interesting. Let's hear it."

"I'd love to. Look, here's the prototype: Dried and chopped weeds in a roll of paper."

"Well, that's a novelty indeed. And what do you do with it?"

"Child's play! You see, the consumer puts one end in his mouth and lights the other. This creates an unpleasant smelling smoke, a mixture of dirty tar, the nerve poison nicotine and other harmful substances, which he then inhales with relish. Obviously, this procedure makes him an enviable, cosmopolitan and cheerful person who, in the eyes of his environment, commands the highest respect and recognition and arouses desire."

"Excuse me, are you out of your mind? You want to tell me that you can find one single fool who is stupid enough to voluntarily burn his money by inhaling the smoke of burnt weeds and paper? Imbeciles, who by choice ruin their health, pollute the environment and claim that they enjoy doing so? Who could think they impress others with this insane behavior? Where on earth are they going to find such disturbed masochists, in a nuthouse?"

"Please leave my office, Mr. Marlboro, I have more important things to do!"

"Have a good day."

This scene is fictional, of course, but: *"How bizarre is this?!"*

The absurd, almost incomprehensible thing is, that it seems as if it actually happened. The triumph of the cigarette around the world has become a reality.

By the way, this scene is a great example of the fact that one should never give up believing in himself and his dreams, no matter how unrealistic they may appear and if others shake their heads.

George Bernard Shaw once put it this way:

"People who think something is impossible should never stand in the way of those who are doing it."

Smoking has no logic. You could laugh tears about Mr. Marlboro's odd business idea. However, it rather makes one cry because it has made the international tobacco industry immensely rich. Therefore, if you smiled about the conversation at the Patent Office, you were amused about yourself. Every smoker has finally fallen for Mr. Marlboro's supposed sales flop.

The allegedly most intelligent creature on this planet has produced one of the most stupid behaviors imaginable.

"Two things are infinite", Albert Einstein is said to have claimed: *"The universe and human stupidity. Although I am not quite sure about the former."*

The billion-dollar cigarette industry is the living proof of Einstein´s frustrating thesis about human brainlessness.

2 to 3 days after the last cigarette:
The sense of taste and smell are flawless again

THIS & THAT ABOUT TOBACCO

Nicotine is the most frequently consumed and freely available addictive substance in our society, next to alcohol. Which is in itself amazing, because nicotine is one of the strongest poisons known to man and one of the most rapidly addictive drugs. Even 50 mg of pure nicotine is lethal to the human body.

To compare how little that is: one sugar cube weighs 3.300 mg (3.3 g). Nicotine in the weight of a single sugar cube would therefore be enough to kill 66 people. Can you imagine the line of 66 people, and in front of it the tiny nicotine cube? Hardly any other poison has such a powerful effect.

Alcoholism is not a "stupid habit", but rather a strongly personality-dependent disease. People who drink liqueur are affected in different ways. Alcohol consumption becomes insidious, and has just as little to do with lack of willpower as dose diabetes. This drug is therefore, in many aspects, different from tobacco. Nevertheless, both are legal substances and they are both hazardous.

One hears time and again that red wine is healthy. That is not true. Certain ingredients of red wine are healthy. However, you can also get these from grape juice. The alcohol in red wine and all other beverages is anything but good for your body.

Tobacco consumption, on the other hand, is a fast-acting substance and it is harmful even in small quantities. And that holds true for *all* human beings. Nicotine has an *immediate* effect on the ganglia of the autonomic nervous system. For these reasons, I believe it is much easier to bury this stinking habit. Cigarettes, once you understand them, are a relatively harmless drug in terms of weaning. At least this has been my personal experience. I know that sounds questionable. Later on, I will explain more in detail why I think so.

For now I can say, that, when I finally stopped smoking, I did not suffer from any physical withdrawal symptoms worth mentioning. At no moment did I drag myself trembling over the floor of a withdrawal cell, shaken by cramps and covered with foam at the mouth, etc.

Cocaine, LSD, Ecstasy, etc. transport the user, at least for a short time, and at lightning speed, into a dazzling world of hallucinations and *"Whow, it's all so colorful here"*. Cigarette smoke, on the other hand, does not trigger any "positive" effects at the beginning. Every newcomer torments himself to become and stay a smoker, so to speak. There is no instant "reward". On the contrary, the first cigarettes cause dizziness, a disgusting burning taste on the tongue, irritation of the throat, and often lead to diarrhea. One has to overcome oneself to get to the next cigarette and that requires some strong mental effort. Only when the persevering person has passed this difficult initial period, does the way stand clear for the permanent degeneration of the smoker's body.

It is precisely this nicotine, a nerve poison in the tobacco plant which works within seconds, that keeps us from throwing in the towel right after the first puff. Since it is the nerves that control our thoughts through the brain, nicotine can manipulate us in this way, *instantly*. Why else would someone be so stupid as to try by hook or crook to develop a taste for something that tastes sooty?

Since each cigarette contains only a tiny dose of nicotine, the effect does not last long. Immediately after smoking one, the nicotine level in the body begins to fall again. The more it sinks, the stronger the desire for the next cigarette. And so it goes, on and on. Finish one cigarette and start another, hour after hour, day after day, year after year, for a lifetime.

Unless you stop smoking.

In the beginning, even the cigarette manufacturers themselves wondered why people could not stop smoking. It was not until the 1970s that it was proven that it was due to the nicotine in the cigarette. This realization caused great joy among the producers on all sides. Hands were shaken, people hugged each other, champagne corks flew and cheers broke out. Then, this knowledge was deliberately locked away and kept secret from the outside world. The fact that cigarettes are toxic was not allowed to be known. The business had become too juicy.

In retrospect, one has to say that they should have been happy to announce that tobacco consumption makes the smoker ill and poisons him with nicotine. Everyone knows this today, but people keep smoking just the same.

With nicotine, everything somehow happens quickly. You get addicted quickly, the effects wear off quickly, and the substance is quickly gone from your body as soon as you stop smoking. It usually takes no more than three to five days for the nicotine to be completely broken down by the body. After that, nothing can be detected. The body has excreted the poison through the kidneys, liver and the bladder or intestines. This is also the reason why smokers so often get cancer of the kidneys, liver, bladder, and intestines. But it must be subtle because this insight does not seem to make many people stop smoking. The smoker does not want to hear warnings and statistics about diseases, premature death, or get well-intentioned advice. All this makes him nervous and prompt him reach for his next cigarette.

Now the question arises, of course, why doesn't the craving for the cigarette subside after five days at the latest? The answer is: because the head still misses the nicotine. After the physical dependence, the psychological dependence comes to the fore. Memory recalls the "beautiful" moments of smoking. People generally tend to repress the negative and remember the good. When it comes to a drug, this behavior is even more pronounced.

Almost unnoticed, an emptiness spreads in the ex-smoker, the feeling of missing something. This is indeed the case. He has banished something from his life with which he had previously spent a large part of his days. And he had found that time of smoking pleasant. So the man who has just given up smoking suppresses the reasons why he wanted to quit, and longs again for his happy time as a smoker. This thinking is about as logical as lifting the 30 km speed limit off the traffic-calmed zone, as no accident has happened for a week, and no child has been run over. So now you can really put your foot down again.

How to say goodbye to addiction forever is the subject of this little booklet. The motto is:

"The one, who knows his enemy, has better chances to defeat him. Even the cigarette has its Achilles heel."

The good news is that just as long as it takes you to

fall for the cigarette, you can also get rid of your greed for it. A good two weeks were enough for me.

After finishing this book, I hope that you too will be on your way to becoming a committed non-smoker. Any craving for a cigarette gone for good. Even if someone smokes in your presence... even if you are consuming alcohol or coffee, feeling stress, anger, boredom, or rage, and even standing in the smokers' corner with your colleagues or sitting at the counter in the smokers' bar; whether you are well or not, you are simply a person who does not need a cigarette. You have become immune. You are an **active** non-smoker, thinking and behaving like someone who never smoked in his life. Like me, you will watch smokers around you, smile and wonder how it was possible that you yourself have ever participated in this utter foolishness.

We are all born with a desires for love, recognition, warmth, food, etc. No human being has ever been born with a craving for nicotine or any other drug. Anyone who smokes has been tempted to do so. By false friends, false role models, or permanent direct and indirect advertising.

The only one who should smoke is the chimney.

At this point, let us take a brief look at the ingredients of "enjoyable" tobacco smoke: *

- Fine dust (tiny particles of dust)
- Carbon monoxide (as in exhaust gases)
- Tar (road surface)
- Nicotine (toxic substance)
- Acetone and toluene (solvent)
- Ammonia (cleaning agents)
- Methanol and benzene (cleaning agents)
- Arsenic and prussic acid (poisons)
- Butane (camping, lighter gas)
- Nickel, cadmium, zinc and lead
- Formaldehyde (disinfectant)
- Methyl isocyanate (chemical)
- Naphtali (pesticide)
- Phenols (pesticide)
- Nitrosamines (toxic nitrogen mixtures)
- Radon and polonium (radioactive)
- Sulphuric acid (chemical product)
- Nitrogen oxides (oxidizing agents)

* Source: State Educational Institute,
  Bremen/Germany

In order to increase the potential for dependency, and to make a cigarette taste more appealing, additives such as sugar, menthol, cocoa, liquorices, honey, and spices or starch, are added. A total of approximately 120 individual substances and 115 mixtures as well as 160 flavors, are offered. In other words, when you puff, you inhale a colorful cocktail of poisons and detergents as well as asphalt and other chemicals. One does it voluntarily, and spends a lot of money on it. Most smokers turn a blind eye to these facts. Instead, a smoker even claims, in all seriousness that the smoke from burning all these disgusting substances tastes delicious.

And because cigarettes seem so irresistible, the smoker is also happy to go along with any price increases without grumbling. Hardly any other product can afford such exorbitant profit margins and tax rates as tobacco. When buying bread in the supermarket, the savings fox thinks hard about whether to take one or the other, because it is 30 cents cheaper. He could save money there. At the checkout, the same person then throws, without batting an eyelid, two Big Boxes on the conveyor belt, which together cost around $20. What is wrong with the smoker? Simple, he's an addict.

Self-deception and irrational behavior are things that smokers have in common with all other drug addicts. For smokers, it is the nicotine in the tobacco, for alcoholics, it is the alcohol in the bottle, and heroin addicts, it is the contents of their syringe.

Why spend a wonderful holiday under the sun once a year, when I can administer myself small doses of this toxic mixture every day for the same money? Can you explain such a thought logically? No? Well, I cannot anymore either. I am going on holiday under the sun.

So what does a smoker who reads this entire negative and horrible information do? Right, usually he reaches for the pack and lights a cigarette. How on earth is that possible? Here is my explanation: The negative information simply does not get through to him. It bounces off something, which was already implemented there before. The area of the brain where they should be perceived and processed is already occupied. *"Sorry amigo, no more room for you here."* If this area was not already blocked, no human would voluntarily smoke. Smoking would probably be more of an alternative torture method.

"Here, smoke this poison stick or tell us where you hid the diamonds".

At school, they showed us teenagers educational videos about lung cancer and smoker's legs. Nowadays, these pictures are printed directly on the front of the box. You do not even have to be able to read. Everywhere you look you're reminded of what you do to yourself if you smoke. Have all these horrifying reports, statistics, warnings, and terribly disgusting images helped to eliminate smoking? Apparently not.

"A passionate smoker, who always reads about the danger of smoking for his health, will in most cases quit... to read."

(Winston Churchill)

A person who imagines that he or she likes to smoke will block out unpleasant stimuli. The "selective perception" of a person, which is necessary for many other areas of life, makes this possible.

According to consciousness research, thousands of sensory impressions are processed in our brain every second. However, we consciously perceive only about 40 of these. If a person were to register all the signals, information and other influences of his environment, he would simply go mad. Our brain just cannot handle all of it. The decisive factor for the smoker is, therefore, not what he knows, sees, senses, or reads, but what he believes. And that is what has made itself comfortable in his brain.

The tobacco industry has been exploiting this fact profitably since its inception. It was already a master in spreading "fake news" when the Internet, Twitter, Instagram and Facebook were still science fiction. Their strategy was, and still is, to constantly feed us with lies and distortions of the truth. "Alternative Truths" is how someone recently named it.

What type of fantasies have been implemented into the smoker's brain:

- *"Smoking relaxes me"*

Have you ever observed a smoker who runs out of cigarettes and has no second pack available? There is no sign of relaxation. A smoker is not relaxed; he is only temporarily not tense. A few seconds after a smoker puts out a cigarette, the nicotine level in his blood starts to drop again. The further it falls, the more uncomfortable he feels and this leads to tension. If this feeling becomes too strong, he puts on his next cigarette and supplies his blood with new nicotine. This goes on all day long. So yes, each cigarette actually gives him the feeling of relaxation, but only for the few minutes of smoking. It is the relaxation of a tension that has slowly built up in him since he put out the previous cigarette. A tension that he would not have had as a non-smoker.

- *"Smoking keeps me awake and increases my concentration"*

Even if it were possible for one and the same substance to relax, awaken and increase concentration, there are better, healthier, and cheaper alternatives for all these states of mind.

It is much more likely to be something like a "placebo effect", a "mental mirage". You feel what you want to feel, but it's not reality.

- *"Smoking is social"*

Most smokers will be likely to confirm this. But ask the non-smokers in your area. They may see things quite differently.

- *"Smoking makes me attractive"*

Sure it does. Brownish discolored teeth, yellow fingers, and foul smelling breath are indeed irresistible. *"What I like most about Frederique are his deep blue eyes and exposed dark yellow tooth necks."*

- *"Smoking tastes good"*

Smoke from soot and tar on the taste buds in the mouth and throat area are the announcers of nicotine. The smoker's body and brain look forward to this. There is no other way to explain why this aroma is perceived as delicious. If the smoker were not addicted, it would be as disgusting to him as it is to any non-smoker.

Only once does a smoker perceive the real taste of cigarette smoke. Namely with the very first cigarette. From the second one on he is already addicted and starts to develop a taste for something that tastes awful.

"I would like three scoops of ice cream in my waffle. One cream-cherry, one mango and one tar-soot."

- *"The cigarette is my little friend. It gives me company and confidence. It's always there for me, wherever I am."*

That's right. The cigarette is a friend, but a fake one. Real friends want you to be well. The cigarette wants the exact opposite. It's a sneaky, evil wolf in sheep's clothing that makes us its slaves. Take a closer look.

- *"Smoking is a reward"*

So is every other drug, for anyone who is an addict to it. Non-addicts can well do without this kind of "premium".

"I smoke because my parents do not want me to"

Sure. They do not want you to cut your thumb off either. Are you doing it anyway, too, you adolescent rebel?

"Smoking makes me feel like I belong."

That is true. But to the wrong group.

If smoking really has all these, literally "fabulous" effects, then why don't all people smoke and why do so many smokers want to quit smoking or have already done so?

About 72 hours after the last cigarette:

All nicotine has disappeared from the body

32

BENEFITS AND ADVANTAGES OF SMOKING

Yes, of course, there are plenty of beneficiaries:

- *"Yay, I can do black zero again. Could it be that maybe I have not set the tobacco tax high enough after all?"* (Federal Minister of Finance)

- *"Ladies and gentlemen. Believe it or not, there are actually people who like to spend more than US$ 10 for a pack of cigarettes. Not in our wildest dreams did we expect this. So let us rejoice at the highest share price ever."* (Shareholders' Meeting at Philip Morris)

- *"Imagine, Mrs. Lannymack. My son got a job as a doctor right away."* (As a specialist for respiratory diseases in oncology).

This list can be continued much further: Advertising- and packaging industry, tobacco growers in third world countries and their underage workforce, logistics companies, private hospitals and nursing homes, pesticide-, pharmaceutical-, nicotine replacement-, cough drop-, airplane smoke detector- and ashtray manufacturers, dentists, cigarette smugglers, tobacco dealers and commodity exchanges, providers of non-smoking seminars, etc.

Millions of people worldwide benefit from the blue haze.

Just think about it… if all the smokers on this planet would give up their moronic habit overnight, thousands and thousands of jobs would be lost. A global stock market crash would shake the markets, as the world has never seen before. This scenario has spawned conspiracy theories that suspect powerful interest groups are in the background to ensure that smokers do not lose the pleasure of their consumption.

So yes, it is very true, there are plenty of beneficiaries. Who you will again look for in vain on the list of profiteers, however, is yourself! Turn and turn it as you like. There are no benefits and advantages for the smoker, unless someone considers it as being positive that he can receive an early disability pension due to the consequences of his addiction.

Imagine that Bill Gates' private secretary knocks on your door one morning and offers a million dollars for your left lung, your liver or at least your tiny little pancreas. Would you say yes? The answer is obvious! Our health makes us a millionaire. We own something we would not sell for all the money in the world. Yet every smoker treats his precious organs like a dump. Open your eyes! Everything related to smoking makes no sense at all.

Conclusion: There are no positive sides to smoking. Searching for them is futile. There is:

- ✓ no use
- ✓ no advantage
- ✓ no improvement
- ✓ no sense
- ✓ no profit
- ✓ no positive effects
- ✓ no positive side effects

Smoking brings the smoker exactly zero point nothing. He only believes it does something for him. He convinces himself and gets it settled into his head.

Not real arguments, but old wives' tales make us reach for a cigarette, cigar, or pipe... fiction instead of facts. Once I had finally opened my eyes, it was a cardboard stick for me to bury this activity.

Read the following paragraphs. Then close your eyes and reflect on what you have read. This is the reality of the false idols implanted in us by the tobacco industry:

- ✓ The good old smoking doctor on the billboard, cheerfully recommending Lucky Strike for being the less irritating cigarette. He is receiving money from the tobacco mafia as well as by curing cigarette related diseases.

✓ The "elegant" Dunhill lady stealthily looking around in the hospital backyard, right by the trash cans. Her skinny, wrinkled neck is adorned with a sinfully expensive diamond necklace. Next to her is an overflowing ashtray, butts and spitted blood all around her. Lacquer black long fingernails glued to mustard yellow fingertips. She is just lighting a cigarette with the previous one. She does not even notice.

✓ Wayne McLaren, the handsome Marlboro cowboy, on his last ride into nirvana. When he is not coughing and choking, he produces croaky sounds through a tube in his throat. He died of lung cancer when he was only 52.

Many people need idols as guiding figures in their lives. Cigarette producers take advantage of this fact. Do not be dazzled. These are well-made illusions that lack any reality. These are lies, subtly inserted into our heads without our noticing.

"One last wish before the firing squad transports you to the afterlife, Lone Rider?"
"Oh yes, a cigarette, please."

Who has not followed this scene in a Lucky Luke comic or in a movie from former times? They make it seem as if cigarettes were the most desirable thing in the world. How silly!

So, during this scene in the film, did you tap yourself on the thighs laughing your head off? Hardly anyone did, although it is obviously hilariously funny and absurd. But bang, without noticing, the lie was nested undetected into your skull.

The cemetery is full of people who thought that smoking was the greatest thing. Lone Rider is now one of many.

Two weeks after the last cigarette:
The mucus in the respiratory tract is clearing up

THE "I SACRIFICE MYSELF METHOD"

Now we are slowly getting to the actual crux of the matter: In what way did I stop smoking and how did this time differ from previous attempts to quit?

The, I call it the **"I sacrifice myself method"**, is used by all those who do not (yet) know how to say, with pleasure, goodbye to the cancer stalk. It is the desolate undertaking to torture oneself to become a non-smoker.

This strategy usually begins with a saying such as: *"Oh well, I guess I will have to start giving up smoking now. I hope I can make it."*

This person believes he must give up something which, at the bottom of his heart, he loves and will miss. He curses himself at the same moment that the resolution is made.

What smoker does not know the following scenario?

"I have decided to quit smoking for good."

"Well, congratulations. I envy you. Do you think you will make it?"

"I hope I will. It is not that easy. However, if you really want something, it will work. It is a question of willpower. Although, it is tough giving up cigarettes forever. Especially the ones I

enjoy most… those in the morning with the delicious coffee and after every meal."

"That's right, those ones taste divine. I myself only really wake up when I hold a coffee and cigarette in my hand."

"Well, it will not be without suffering. You are not going to see me at any parties for a while. I am sure I will be unmotivated, stressed and irritable for a while. I don't want you to have to deal with that."

"Of course, I understand. That is very kind of you. Alcohol without a cigarette, that is an absolute no go. But I'm sure you'll get there eventually."

"Thanks, I hope so too."

"Come on, let's share the last Chesterfield, buddy. Tomorrow is your big day."

This person means well. But good intentions are not the same as doing well. They are the opposite of being good. This fellow wants to get off the drug, but he is taking the wrong approach.

With the "I sacrifice myself approach", the well-meaning fellow assumes that:

> ✓ He is facing the worst withdrawal symptoms. *This scares him.*
>
> ✓ He will in future renounce something desirable that has given him pleasure so far. *He does not want that.*

✓ He is embarking on a long and painfully boring journey of privation. *That puts him off.*

To be honest, this approach is hardly going to work. In my opinion, symptoms such as lack of motivation, stress, mood swings, restlessness, fatigue, irritability, etc. can also be brought on. Self-fulfilling negative scenarios make no sense. They produce expectations about states of mind that have not yet occurred and may never happen. Stay positive! Nothing like this has seriously happened to me. And even if some of them had occurred, they were only temporary.

Smokers who torment themselves with the "I sacrifice myself method" to stop smoking, like to use the fairy tale of "habit" as an excuse. *"How incredibly hard is it to let go of something I have done for so long."*

Smokers who, like me, become non-smokers with the "Lead-motive method", manage to get rid of this habit in a relatively relaxed manner, and it happens almost immediately. Why? For the same reason that they get used to the new car, getting up later, falling in love, promotion at work or start using reading glasses. Simply because they are aware that they will benefit from it.

The "I sacrifice myself method" rarely converts anyone into a real non-smoker for the long term. At best, it turns the smoker into an inactive smoker. One, who temporarily stops smoking, even though he would like to. That's why he has to think about it permanently. He does not even believe in his own intentions. However, a firm belief in success is one of the basic requirements for winning the game.

The person, who forces and "sacrifices" himself, has not stopped. He has only put himself into "standby mode" for the moment. He is like a "sleeper", who can awaken at any moment from his self-imposed, nightmarish self-flagellation. Then it takes less than 5 seconds until the lighter clicks and the bad conscience in him begins to giggle.

His "sleep" can last hours, days, weeks, but also years. Still, it always remains a laborious fight against windmills. A stable permanent state looks different. The remorsefully sacrificing fellow is nothing more than a ticking time bomb that can explode at any time. He not only looks like a fuse, he has one and is just waiting to strike the match.

So, what usually "liberates" the "poor suffering victim" from his "martyrdom"? Here are a few examples:

> ✓ A special moment: *"Well done, now I have earned myself a "nice tasty" cigarette after such a long abstinence."*

✓ A tragic moment: *"Never mind, I can smoke again. Everything is going down the drain anyway."*

✓ Fake friends: *"Listen, now that you've been a non-smoker for so long, a single cigarette won't hurt you. Come on, I'll give you a fag."* Drug addicts are afraid of losing a "companion". It makes them look like a weakling and puts them in need of an explanation for their behavior. It imposes the unpleasant pressure on them, to also try quitting, which they do not want to. So they would rather seduce the person who managed to quit.

✓ Anger or stress: *"It's driving me crazy! Where's my tranquilizing cigarette?"* Smoking reduces the perceived stress only during the few minutes in which the smoker smokes his cigarette. For the rest of his existence, a smoker, just as all drug addicts, is under permanent (withdrawal) stress. This is caused by the desire for the next dose.

✓ Frustration about something or someone: *"Oh well, that's what he/she gets from it now. It's his/her fault that I've relapsed."*

Inactive smokers using the "I sacrifice myself method", are back on the "drip" from the very first cigarette. Even if they had compulsively managed to stay smoke-free for years before. They were simply non-smoking smokers all that while, not truly non-smokers. There is a huge difference. How could it be otherwise, since they never really got "clean"?

Those who "sacrifice" their smoking habit usually feel an urge for a replacement, although this is not justified. Replacement is only needed for something we miss. Something, which leaves a vacuum to be filled. Nobody needs to inhale toxic dirty smoke when you think about it. Therefore, its departure has actually left no vacuum. It's a mindset. You just have to let it go. That is all there is to it.

What is perceived as emptiness is not a loss but a gain. It is the newly granted time. He who smokes 20 cigarettes for 5 minutes each, wastes about 1.5 hours a day. This time is given back to him as soon as he stops smoking. This is precious time that can be used for other things in life. You can relax more often, devote more time to yourself and to your partner, family or friends, or you can finally do what you didn't have time for before.

Anyone who tells himself that, as a non-smoker, he now suddenly has to constantly stuff chocolate and cream cakes inside himself is barking up the wrong tree. This behavior serves at best to prepare an excuse to start puffing again at the first possible moment.

"Of course Thomas, if I had been you I would have continued smoking too, with 7 kg weight gain in 12 weeks. We understand you. It is all good."

My personal experience is completely different. A short time after I stopped smoking, my eating habits changed. Chocolate and other desserts attracted me less and less. Even the desire for meat diminished. Instead of Bolognese sauce, I began to prefer more subtle flavors such as spaghetti with pesto or with olive oil and garlic. I bought a blender and began to prepare delicious fruit juice smoothies. Self-mixed muesli found access to my breakfast options. Instead of beer, I developed a preference for wine on special occasions. For the first time in my life, I ordered a Caesar salad as my main course in a restaurant, simply because I felt the desire for it. In my smoking days, salad was not a food for me, rather an unwanted side dish included in the meal.

I eat only twice a day. A late breakfast and an early dinner. Chips, salt sticks and other nibbles do not tempt me. Instead, I love to eat fresh fruit between meals. Since I feel fitter, I also move more. As a smoker, I preferred the comfortable resting mode. This way my body burnt far fewer calories.

A person who practices the "Lead-motive method" does not need a substitute, because he does not miss anything. If someone gains extreme weight after stopping smoking, it is because he regrets the loss of the cigarette and compensates the sad feeling of emptiness with increased food intake. These are often sweets and other unhealthy snacks. He eats out of self-pity and boredom.

Not smoking anymore turned my life completely upside down. Finally, I can enjoy culinary delights. Eating is no longer the annoying occupation before the cigarette.

I even became a passionate sporty person. Almost every morning, before breakfast, I go out in a canoe to the swimming platform. From there I jump into the river and enjoy ploughing through the water. In former times, I would have smoked at least three cigarettes during this time, accompanied by half a liter of coffee with lots of sugar, and would be sitting on a chair. Now I can literally feel how my lung volumes slowly expand. The oxygen finds its way through previously sooty airways. Newly created energy can be felt in my body every day.

Not long ago I woke up in the morning already tired and caught myself yawning in the late afternoon. Lack of oxygen was responsible for it. Such symptoms disappeared when I stopped smoking. What a wonderful experience. A medically experienced friend explained the reason for this to me: Oxygen and carbon monoxide (from tobacco smoke) compete for the docking sites of the red blood cells. This race has come to an end in my body, thank God! Better full steam than full of steam.

"Oh well, I guess I will have to start giving up smoking now. I hope I can make it."

That is nonsense. You do not start quitting eating either. Quitting happens in the moment, as it does when you put out your last cigarette.

From the second week after the last cigarette:

Cilia cleans themselves of soot

COMPENSATORY SATISFACTION
AND OTHER HOKEY POKEY

Good idea! Just yet again not for the person who really wants to quit smoking.

For quite a while now, the market for substitute products for cigarette consumption has been flourishing. Guess who produces most of these "saviors", and earns a lot of money with them. That's right, Mr. Marlboro's grandchildren.

These "saviors" are the result of the demand of all inactive "smoke victims" for a replacement crutch. Those who actually do become a non-smoker with them will achieve the non-smoking goal despite and not because of these replacements. A real, active non-smoker can easily do without them. E-cigarettes, nicotine chewing gums and patches, water pipes, etc. are primarily beneficial to the person who manufactures and sells them. Poison with the taste and smell of strawberries, *"how delicious is that!"* Promoted and sold like this, the inhibition threshold is not very high.

No one needs a substitute for an evil. Just be glad to be rid of it. Replacing the nicotine (of the cigarette) with nicotine (from another source) seems about as sensible as giving up cigarettes by smoking cigars.

You probably wouldn't advise an alcoholic to stop, by nibbling brandy chocolates either, would you?

The nicotine has to get out of the body to end the physical addiction. This is prevented by substitute products such as patches, chewing gum, etc. As a matter of fact, they are not substitutes at all, but the same addictive poison, only in a different dosage and form. So, they are not a good idea. The best substitute for nicotine is no nicotine.

In the case of a drug that causes severe physical withdrawal symptoms, such as heroin, a substitute may be temporarily useful. But with a cigarette? No! Don't be foolish. Do not trade cholera for the plague. If substitutes were really necessary, how would I and many others have made the jump without them?

Drugs and nicotine substitutes should be used only as part of professional withdrawal therapy wherein, when properly applied, they can break the behavioral automatisms, and simultaneously carry out a successive drug withdrawal. The e-cigarette, however, is never used, because the procedure of holding something and sucking on it is too similar to actually smoking and will thereby conserve the habit.

Did you know that there are now also some great apps for smartphones that allow you to follow the progress of your smoking cessation? They show you exactly and at any moment, how many cigarettes you have *not* smoked, what benefit you have achieved and how much money you have saved… right down to the second decimal place. Even the additional life span you have gained is calculated to the minute. And, of course, all this can be shared with the rest of the world three times a day via an Instagram-link. Isn't that amazing?!

Indeed, it is. From my point of view, as amazingly superfluous as with the substitutes we've discussed. Again, in the end, everyone, *except* the user of the app benefits. By keeping the cigarette front and center through its constant presence on the display of their phone, it retains its place of prominence in their life. This is not very smart, in my opinion. When you part with something, you have a reason for it. So do it and forget about it. Erase picture and name of your former "love" from the display and from your mind.

Every time you check on your app to see how many days you have been smoke-free, the cigarette appears in this train of thought. Free yourself mentally from everything that reminds you of your dark past. You are a non-smoker now, and non-smokers do not need to think about cigarettes ever. What counts is your future and it starts now, nicotine-free. Erase from your mind thoughts of the drug! Do not talk about it, and do not think about it. There are much more important things and more useful apps with which to occupy yourself with.

In my previous attempts to quit smoking, long before smartphones and apps had even been invented, I had stuck the last pack to the wall. Next to it, I attached a board on which I kept a tally sheet for every day of not smoking. It looked somewhat like an altar and in the same way was a sad reminder which didn't help me a bit. It gave me the feeling of a prisoner in a cell, waiting to be released soon. Again, I felt I was a "victim".

2 to 12 weeks after the last cigarette:

The lungs are cleared of mucus and soot particles

THE "LEAD-MOTIVE METHOD"

My bladder tumor diagnosis was not the deciding factor in my quitting smoking in record time.

Let us not fool ourselves. No one has to wait for the bad news to come in. In some cases it may help build up the necessary motivation. However, then it is usually too late. The incorrigible one may even show a defiant reaction:

"Now more than ever, it's too late to stop anyway."

Who has not heard stories of people with progressive bronchitis, COPD or even the first signs of cancer and the like, who continue to smoke as they did before. Some people will give up eating rather than give up smoking. Such behavior is completely unreasonable.

But be careful: If you are a non-smoker, you should not judge this kind of acting too lightly, just because you cannot understand the destructive behavior. Nicotine is a drug. Any smoker, who does not find the right mental approach to confront it, will actually find it extremely difficult to quit. I speak from personal experience.

Psychology explains the illogical conduct of a person, in this case the smoker, as "cognitive dissonance": The thinking does not fit the behavior. It is case of doing something that my logic refutes as completely stupid. Colloquially, this behavioral disorder is known as "self-cheating". It engenders a conflict that needs to be resolved. The brain hates these kinds of states. Consequently, the cigarette lover looks for excuses and pretexts to justify his attitude towards his conscience. The longer he smokes, the greater the dissonance. Smoking is an emotional decision, not a logical one. And against emotions, logic has little chance in the first place. It is about the same as the feeling of being in love.

As mentioned before, I had also made several serious attempts before, to avoid the smog from the paper tube. Each time I failed, because my approach was the wrong one. Or was I just not strong enough? Am I a wimp? No!

If willpower would be the key, then only weak-willed people would smoke and strong-willed people would quit right away. But that's not the case. Look at smokers. Many are very successful, highly intelligent and self-confident people from all social classes of society. Thus, being strong-willed is obviously no guarantee of success in quitting smoking.

My bladder tumor diagnosis however, did make me think more intensively. And so I remembered the marketing lectures of my business studies from almost forgotten days. What had I been taught at that time about consumer behavior?: *"Man as a consumer is not rational. That is why he is so willing to be pulled in front of the cart by clever advertising."*

The tobacco industry is a master of these indoctrination activities, as the foregoing meeting at the Patent Office illustrated. As absurd as this anecdote may sound, it has become reality. Thanks to direct and subtle advertising messages, the clever Mr. Marlboro succeeded over time in associating the cigarette with attributes such as adventure, independence, relaxation, self-confidence and coziness. Even the erotic version of the "cigarette after" is internalized by the smoker. None of this is true, of course. It is all lies. And yet, they have found their way into the smoker's upstairs room, and without criticism.

By now, everyone knows that the smoking cool guys and sensual women in the cinema, on TV and on advertising posters, or the Camel logo on the racing car are no coincidence. Neither is the fact that cigarettes are always displayed at the cash register so that everyone really *has to* notice them.

All this exposure costs the cigarette manufacturers vast sums of money. And they are only too happy to invest, because subliminal advertising is, by far, more effective and therefore the most lucrative payback per dollar. The subliminal message is not consciously noticed, and there is no way to defend yourself against it. One cannot protect oneself from something that is not actually perceived. This is how cruel cigarette advertising works.

After I reconsidered the content of my marketing lectures again, I recognized that I was not defenselessly at the mercy of these practices, because I could see them for what they were. I could realize the part that they played in the formation of the senseless habit. It illuminated for me how we humans tend to hide unwanted information. This behavior is a key point. Exactly there, I figured out in that moment of clarity, where I had to start in order to free myself from my dependence.

What is decisive, for people in general, and the smoker in particular, is not just what he knows, but mainly what has settled in his subconscious. These form what he believes and recalls, whether it is the truth or a lie. And a lie, repeated often enough, eventually becomes the truth. Especially if it comes in handy for the recipient.

My new and successful approach was to beat the enemy with his own weapons. I asked myself:

How can I fight back? Quite simply, I must repeat the truth so often that it suppresses the untruth and cements itself as reality. I had to turn the tables.

So I formulated a credo for myself, which I would use from now on, when the lie reoccurs in my head. It says:

"There is absolutely no reason to smoke… not one. I'm a non-smoker. I am strong, healthy, active, full of joie de vivre and energy. I will not poison my body with stinky nicotine or smear it with slimy tar. No, I'm not that stupid!"

At first I read my credo from a piece of paper that I always carried in my pocket. I repeated it at every opportunity… on the bus, on the park bench, in the queue at the bank counter, even on the toilet.

- ✓ Control your thoughts, and then you control your life.
- ✓ If your previous thoughts do not bring you to your goal, change your thoughts.
- ✓ If you always behave in the same way, you should not expect different results.

Based on these assumptions the "Lead-motive method" could be developed. The name "Lead-motive" is my variation of the expression "Leader Wolf". The leader dominates, and leads his pack. My lead-motive became the leader of my thoughts. Also crucial to my approach is that man cannot have two thoughts at the same time. Here lies another key to the success of the "Lead-motive method".

Have you ever heard of the following story? It is about the conversation between an American Indian and his son:

"Daddy, why is man sometimes good and sometimes bad?"

"Look, we each have two wolves inside of us", replied the father. *"One gray and one white. The gray wolf wants evil, the white wolf wants good." Both are in a constant battle against each other."*

"And which of the two wins?" the child asks after a while of consideration?

"The one you feed the most, my son."

If we apply this thoughtful and wise story to the theme of this book, it is the gray wolf that encourages us to smoke. I have succeeded in making the white wolf in me invincible. He got all the food. That was the whole trick.

The process of smoking always follows the same pattern. As soon as the nicotine level has fallen below a certain level, the desire for the next cigarette awakens. This causes the automatic grab for the pack. A few seconds pass between these two steps. This gap is the moment when we have to become active. It requires all our concentration. In the beginning more, later the effort diminishes. This slot, one must fill by repeating the credo and feeding the white wolf with the truth. Remember that the first three to five days after the last cigarette will take some getting used to.

It is the time the body needs to get rid of all nicotine. Quickly the gray wolf appears and demands supplies. This is unavoidable, because your body is deprived of a drug it has been used to for a long time. But let us be honest to ourselves. Is that really so impossible to bear? Does it hurt terribly? No, it is just a brief flash of desire. You will come through it without harm. Withstand this short span of time and the already weakening withdrawal symptoms will subside rapidly. No one has ever died from nicotine withdrawal. You won't either ;-).

Do not succumb to the worry that you will miss something, relapse or not make it. Don't let that feeling paralyze you. Overcoming fears is one of the greatest challenges in life. Accept them, do not hide from them. Remember how often you have been afraid of something new in your life... your first day at school, riding your bike without help, your driving test, your new job or your first kiss. And aren't we all happy and grateful not to have given in to these fears?

Are you still afraid? Well, then do it with fear. What's the problem? Each of us is constantly deciding what to do with our lives. You must not shirk or avoid responsibility. Not making a decision is a decision in itself, but it's usually the wrong one.

Those who have relapsed, by the way, have not failed. They only fail, when they stop trying, when they resign and throw in the towel. So far, the willing person has at least already found out how it doesn't work. Now he just has to keep trying until he finds the way that finally leads him to his goal.

You, dear reader, are lucky to have gotten to know the "Lead-motive method". If you use it correctly, it will lead you directly and without much trying into a drug-free life. Get ready. Celebrate defeating your ridiculous enemy and experience the joyous victory of starving him out once and for all. Welcome and enjoy the test of strength with this basically toothless calf-biter in the absolute certainty that you are stronger. **You are!** The gray wolf is only the temporary harbinger of your future independence. He will disappear if you ignore him.

How did my three days of nicotine withdrawal go? I could feel the gray wolf inside me getting nervous. He was running out of "food" and began to rebel. Instead of whispering as before, his tone became louder. I held out. On the fourth day, I could feel his weakness building up. Nevertheless, every now and then moments came when he seemed to gather his last strength to make my life difficult. Since I knew that these would be his last twitches, it was easy for me to stand up to him by constantly "praying" my credo. The desire for a cigarette during the first three to five days comes suddenly. The gray wolf flashes up and he is so strong and deceitful that he makes the grip for the cigarette an impulse. In these moments, I knew that I had to focus in order to resist the temptation. I realized that when I withstood the first impulse, the languish lasts a few minutes at a time and then quickly loses intensity. In this short time frame, I kept repeating my credo, remembering why I wanted to stop smoking. I also told myself short, plain and clear mantras like:

"Cigarette smoke is dirt, toxic dirt. I'm not gonna smear my body with it."

Inside, I imagined myself lighting a cigarette. With this thought, I formulate mantras like:

"What I do is absolutely ridiculous. Smoking dried weeds with paper is just stupid. No, I do not want to belong to that group of people. I never wanted; I was seduced to do it. Now I decide for myself."

Anyone can give free rein to his or her imagination when it comes to the wording of mantras. Use the passages in the book you have marked. It is only important that you speak these sentences/mantras and the credo internally. In this way you prevent the lies of the past from spreading. Now it says again, *"Sorry amigo, there is no place for you here."* But this time it is the good one who has spread and settled.

The decisive thing is to have these kinds of positive thoughts, so that the gray wolf cannot appear, expanding his lies in your head. Remember, one can only have one thought at a time. My credo and mantras helped me to survive the greed that lasted only a few minutes, when I would normally have smoked a cigarette and felt bad afterwards. I knew that I was going to win. **And I won!**

You think not smoking for three days is difficult? Then try not to complain, criticize or bitch about others for three days, not once, then you know what difficult means. Both of these three-day-exercises, quitting smoking and quitting pointing at others, make sense and both change your life, and that of your fellow human beings, in a very positive way.

***

Then the dreamlike time of reward began. After only a few weeks, I noticed the first positive changes.

As a smoker, I was reluctant to the stairs up to higher floors, but then I suddenly started to enjoy it. Instead of using an elevator, escalator or tediously dragging myself up step by step to gasp for air, I now literally flew up there. What an unforgettable experience when I arrived at the top for the first time and thought, *"Strange, it feels so good, where is the sense of shortness of breathing, I used to experience?"* Me, who not so long ago was still whistling when I breathed and felt breathing difficulties even at the slightest effort. Me, who is slowly approaching 60 years of age. How can it be that every day makes me feel more vital?

I had another aha-experience with dental care. A couple of weeks after I had stopped smoking, I noticed a pleasant change when brushing my teeth. When rinsing, there was no more blood to be seen, and the nausea I had had when I brushed with the toothbrush far back in my mouth, had disappeared. A condition to which I had become accustomed, unnoticed, as a heavy smoker. My body recovered internally and externally. You could literally see it in my face. Even the complexion of my skin began to regenerate. I only noticed it when friends mentioned it.

Now that I have stopped smoking, I drink less coffee. I used to think that cigarettes and coffee belonged together like Tom and Jerry. In my new life as a non-smoker, my caffeine consumption has been greatly reduced. It is mostly limited to the good morning coffee, and now and then too an espresso in the afternoon. I find myself looking for herbal and fruit teas, when shopping. Who would have thought it? Me, of all people, who had hardly wasted any time on healthy food and lifestyle. Something had happened to me, activated by the simple fact that I stopped smoking. The rediscovered vitality had awakened in me the desire for "more". More strength and more endurance, more lust for life, more condition, more, more, more… Living healthy became a philosophy that has enriched my life extremely, ever since. My revived sense of taste constantly discovers new and almost forgotten pleasures. These are real pleasures, not imaginary ones like the dirty stinking smoke of the poisonous smoldering stalks. In one sentence: I am simply in a better shape. Physically and mentally.

Also, the urge to do something at least every hour of the day, namely to smoke a cigarette, has disappeared. This gives me a new feeling of freedom. Before that I was a prisoner of my "pleasurable" addiction.

Every now and then, I still noticed twitches of the slowly starving gray wolf, until one day they simply stopped. It lasted altogether only a few weeks. In the beginning he was emaciated and weakened, but not dead. But every hour, every day without nicotine, he became more and more sickly, slowly but surely withering away through the "food deprivation".

Nevertheless, I remained vigilant. He does not give up so easily. He's an old, cunning wolf. On some days, he suddenly picks up speed again, and out of nowhere he makes himself felt for an instant. Without warning the thought of a cigarette flashes up. With me it was on the 9th and 14th day. Then it was finally over. With the "I sacrifice myself method" that I had practiced before, this last rebellion was enough to drive me back into its clutches. I became weak, could not resist, was even grateful for the temptation. Afterwards I felt miserable, called myself a failure. The frustration and disappointment were the cause for the next cigarette, then another one. And all of a sudden I was an active smoker again.

With the "Lead-motive method" it went differently. I noticed the gray wolf rearing up...

... and smiled.

I did not mind at all anymore. Automatically, the "real pictures", connected with my credo, appeared before my inner eye. The attack of the skinny gray wolf that had just begun disappeared as quickly as it had appeared.

In the original manuscript of this book, at this point, I suggested, that one should also think of one's fellow men. How they can benefit and what they can be spared if you stop smoking. One of my test readers however, wrote me that this was not a good idea. She is right. Firstly, because every smoker has heard these recommendations already x times. Secondly, because they're not a real motivation. They merely suggest a guilty conscience. If you want to quit smoking, or whatever else you wish to get rid of, you must do it for yourself. Resolutely, voluntarily, and of your own accord. A smoker who forces himself to give up for the good of others also remains a "victim". A negative trying to inform a positive, and that never lasts.

With these thoughts in mind, I remembered a quote I had read a long time ago and it stuck with me. It is also by the Irish playwright George Bernard Shaw:

"He who begins to sacrifice himself for the people he loves will end up hating them."

I do not want to expose you to this danger. Remember better what kind of person you wanted to be for yourself before you started smoking. Becoming a smoker was definitely not one of your life goals. Ask yourself if the child you once were would be proud of you today. If you quit smoking for yourself, everyone around you will automatically benefit from it as well. Think of non-smoking as a free wellness treatment for your body. At the same time, it is one of the most valuable gifts you can give yourself.

"I will start by cutting down smoking. That is a big step forward after all. Peter only smokes at the coffee party, Paul only on vacation, and Mary has been smoking exactly five

cigarettes a day, always at the same time of day, for several years. She is convinced that her body is able to process five cigarettes a day without leaving any residues that could harm her."

You want my opinion? Strike Grandpa Gotho, Winston Churchill, Peter, Paul and Mary from your thoughts. For the same reasons that were explained at the beginning of this book. These people belong to a rare species and are extremely endangered.

So, enough of the long speech. *"The march of a thousand kilometers begins with the first step,"* says an Asian wisdom.

In that sense:

All the best and enjoy your walk in and through a second life...

9 months after the last cigarette:

                      The lungs begin to cleanse completely

EPILOG

I have been living in Central America for over 20 years now. Here, the cigarette has basically been "out of fashion" for a long time. The youth in these countries are very health-conscious and enthusiastic about sports. I had assumed that in Europe this trend would also be noticeable, by now.

When I flew across the Atlantic again for the first time in many years to work for a few months in the south of France, I was shocked. So many people, especially young ones, who smoke, male and female. I would not have expected that. The cigarette has become chic and socially acceptable again.

One difference with the past, however, is that today there are always some users of e-cigarettes in every group. I am afraid that this could become the new trend, or rather, be pushed into being a trend by the nicotine mafia.

With me, this topic is fortunately an issue of the past. I hope it will be with you soon.

***

Congratulations! You have read this book to the end. How do you feel? Did my story inspire you?

Make the credo your habit too. It can become your guide for a second, liberated life:

"There is absolutely no reason to smoke… not one. I'm a non-smoker. I am strong, healthy, active, full of joie de vivre and energy. I will not poison my body with stinky nicotine or smear it with slimy tar. No, I'm not that stupid!"

Carry this little booklet with you and, whenever you feel like it, open it at any page, and read a few paragraphs. It is not a pocketbook for nothing. It is meant to accompany you.

Here are the **cornerstones** of the method I used, summed up again. As I said in the beginning, repetition is decisive:

By constantly repeating lies, the cigarette could gain access to you. Through the constant repetition of truth, it will be driven out again.

Lighting minced weeds in a roll of paper at one end to inhale the toxic smoke on the other, is embarrassing, ridiculous, pointless and stupid. Observe the smokers in your environment very closely. In the street café, in the park, at the bus stop, in the smokers' corner in front of the hospital entrance or wherever you discover one. Does it really look cool and casual? Take a look in the mirror while you are smoking and you will see what I am trying to explain to you.

Gray wolf - white wolf: Nobody can have two thoughts at the same time. Determine for yourself whether to "feed" addiction or insist on freedom.

For a long time, the white wolf in you has been barely perceptible. When it was weak and afraid, it crept away somewhere. The gray wolf dominated and controlled your thoughts of a habitual smoker at will. Right now, he is even stronger than you are. **You** have to let the white wolf grow and become stronger.

It will take you a few days to nurture the white wolf inside you. Give him all the "food" from now on, then the roles will change quickly. Protect the good wolf with your true thoughts. Then it is the bad wolf that must retreat in hunger. For the first three to five days, you deprive him of both, nicotine and your attention. Hold on, you can do it. When the gray wolf comes into your thoughts, ignore him. Tell him you're busy today. Maybe tomorrow. Then feed the white wolf and listen to his good advice. If it worked for me, why not for you?

Don't be afraid of withdrawal symptoms. Many non-smokers find out in retrospect that their panic before rehab was much worse than the rehab itself. Look forward to it and enjoy it, especially the first, exciting days when the nicotine leaves your body. Perceive it consciously. Experience it like an adventure, out of the monotonous gray and nebulous routine and into a new, wonderful life. The short phase of withdrawal is the "sad" end of your smoking life and the beginning of your regained freedom.

Withdrawal symptoms are a (good) sign that your body is reacting and defending itself. It fights against nicotine withdrawal and slowly but surely breaks down the remaining poison. Soon the accompanying symptoms are gone forever. Then you are a non-smoker, as if you had never needed a cigarette in your life.

So look forward to the appearance of the gray wolf. Realize how harmless and small he really is. He won't like your confident reaction. Suddenly you're in control. He's never seen anything like it with you.

Although it should be self-evident, I will mention it at the very end anyway: You can read this book and twenty others about quitting smoking, be hypnotized or injected, attend non-smoking seminars and get a prescription from the doctor for "Champix". **All this will not transform you into an active non-smoker if you do not really and frankly want to be, or if you are afraid of losing something.** Nicotine is not an opponent that you can knock out listlessly.

The first step in a non-smoking life is to make a joyful agreement with yourself, and then get going.

A good moment to do so and start is **now**, since you have just read so much negative and nothing positive about smoking. Not tomorrow, or next Monday, or when all your problems are solved, or if you spit blood, or your wife is pregnant, or on January 1st. Life is too short for "sometime". Look forward to the fact that you will smell better, feel healthier, vital, strong and free. You will have more time and be in better shape. Enjoy that food and drinks taste right again, that you are free from the compulsions of addiction, that your body regenerates etc. and that you have more money for the really enjoyable things in life.

Ask yourself, *"Do I really want to stop poisoning myself?"* Your answer is, ***"of course I do."***

Are you ready? **Of course you are!** Otherwise, you wouldn't have read this book. Nobody reads a book about not smoking just for the fun of it. So come on, now's the time! What have you got to lose? Smoking's not great. Not smoking is great!

For many decisions in your life, at the moment you make them, you don't know if you are right or wrong. If you decide to become a non-smoker, you can be one hundred percent sure that you are doing the right thing. Ban cigarettes, lighters and ashtrays from your life. As of today, you no longer need any of that stuff.

You are a confident, strong and enjoyable person in your non-smoker freedom! Be proud of yourself. It's in your hands, you decide.

Robert G. Ingersoll put it this way:

"Happiness is not a reward, it is a consequence.
Suffering is not a punishment, it is a result."

***

If you like, write me your impressions and experiences with this "guide", which actually is not supposed to be one. Could this reading motivate you to follow my example? For me your feedback is welcomed information, hopefully a confirmation of my efforts. Who knows? I would be happy to hear from you:

kontakt@grenzenlos-peter-kruse.com

A short review from you on Amazon would be a valuable gift for me and for all those people who want to quit smoking, looking for references and examples to follow. So if I have been able to help you, please take just 10 minutes and leave a small review for all those who are looking for help.

Thank you very much!

ABOUT THE AUTHOR

Peter Kruse spent 40 years as a happy smoker. Today he lives as a happy non-smoker. The difference is that he no longer spends a fortune to continuously supply his body with small amounts of poison, which permanently worsened his quality of life.

"My Gift to help you quit smoking" is his second book.

www.**instagram**.com/peter.kruse.autor

For 10 years, he has lived on the beautiful Rio Dulce, near the Caribbean coast of Guatemala. If you want to, you can visit him here:

www.casa-perico.com

Printed in Great Britain
by Amazon